MW00390193

MARBLE NOTEBOOK

This Book Belongs To:

....

Made in the USA
Middletown, DE
03 March 2020

85686401R00060